DIY EYEBROW SHAPING AND MAINTENANCE TECHNIQUES

Master the Art of Perfect Brows at Home with Expert Tips and Tricks

VINCE WALTER

DISCLAIMER

This book's content is only meant to be used for general informative purposes. Although the author has taken great care to ensure the content is accurate and thorough, no warranties or assurances on the information's accuracy, correctness, or reliability are provided. It is recommended that readers employ their own judgment and discretion when applying any material found in this book to their particular situation.

The information in this book is not intended to replace professional advice, nor is the author an expert in any of the subjects covered. It is recommended that readers consult with experienced professionals regarding any particular issues or concerns.

Any name that may be mentioned or referred in this book does not imply endorsement, recommendation, or relationship on the part of the author with any person, entity, good, website, or association. These references are made only for informational purposes and are not meant to be taken as recommendations or endorsements.

The information contained in this book may cause readers to suffer loss or damage, for which the author disclaims all obligation and accountability. The only people accountable for the decisions and actions taken by readers using the information presented are themselves.

Any names, characters, companies, locations, activities, occasions, and incidents referenced in this book are either made up or the result of the author's imagination. Any likeness to real people, living or dead, or to real things is entirely coincidental.

This book's content may change at any time, without prior notice, according to the author.

The onus is on the reader to verify whether there have been any updates or revisions.

The reader accepts the conditions of this disclaimer by reading this book. Please do not read this book or use its contents if you do not agree to these terms.

Table of Contents

CHAPTER 1

UNDERSTANDING EYEBROW ANATOMY

The Structure of Eyebrows: Hair Growth Patterns and Cycles

Eyebrows are made up of thousands of tiny hair follicles, each playing a distinct role in forming the brow's unique shape and texture. These hairs follow a specific growth pattern: growing upwards near the inner brow, arching outward at the peak, and angling downward at the tail. This directional growth creates the natural contour that defines the brow's character. Understanding these growth patterns is crucial for effective shaping and maintenance, as it allows for adjustments that retain the natural flow.

The eyebrow hair growth cycle consists of three main phases: **anagen (growth phase), catagen (transition phase)**, and **telogen (resting phase)**. During the anagen phase, new hair grows actively from the follicle, which can last several weeks. In the catagen phase, the hair stops growing, and the follicle shrinks, a process lasting about 2-3 weeks. Finally, during the telogen phase, which lasts several months, the hair rests before naturally shedding and being replaced by new growth. This cycle ensures eyebrows maintain their thickness and fullness over time. Factors such as genetics, age, and overall health can influence hair density and regrowth, highlighting the importance of tailored eyebrow care.

Types of Eyebrow Shapes and How They Complement Facial Features

Eyebrow shapes are as unique as the individuals they adorn, and their style can significantly enhance or alter one's facial appearance. Common eyebrow shapes include **arched, straight, rounded, and S-shaped brows**, each bringing distinct effects to the face. Arched brows, for example, are known for adding definition and lifting the overall facial structure, making them a popular choice for those with rounder faces. Straight brows lend a softer, more natural look, often complementing oval or long faces by creating balance.

Rounded brows are ideal for softening angular features, making them suitable for square or rectangular face shapes. S-shaped brows, which curve gently before tapering at the tail, add complexity and drama to facial expressions, working well for heart-shaped or diamond-shaped faces. The key to selecting the right shape lies in considering natural brow lines, bone structure, and personal aesthetic preferences. A well-chosen eyebrow shape can enhance natural beauty by framing the eyes and harmonizing facial proportions.

The Role of Eyebrows in Facial Symmetry and Expressions

Eyebrows are pivotal in defining facial symmetry and conveying emotions, making them one of the most expressive features of the face. Symmetry is often associated with attractiveness, and balanced eyebrows contribute significantly to this perception. Uneven brows can disrupt harmony, drawing attention away from the eyes and other facial features. Symmetry doesn't necessarily mean identical brows, but they should align in height, arch, and length to complement the face evenly.

Beyond symmetry, eyebrows play a central role in non-verbal communication. They help convey emotions such as surprise, anger, curiosity, or joy through subtle movements. Raised brows can indicate shock or interest, while furrowed brows suggest concentration or displeasure.

These nuances in expression are essential for interpersonal interactions, making eyebrow grooming a tool not just for beauty but for enhancing social communication. Proper maintenance ensures eyebrows remain expressive and balanced, reinforcing their vital role in framing the face.

CHAPTER 2

TOOLS AND EQUIPMENT FOR EYEBROW SHAPING

Essential Tools: Tweezers, Scissors, Razors, and More

To achieve precise and well-shaped eyebrows at home, having the right tools is critical. **Tweezers** are the cornerstone of eyebrow grooming, allowing for the removal of stray hairs with accuracy. High-quality tweezers with slanted or pointed tips provide a better grip and reduce the risk of breakage. For beginners, slanted-tip tweezers are easier to handle, while pointed-tip tweezers excel in removing finer hairs.

Eyebrow scissors are essential for trimming unruly or overgrown brow hairs. Opt for a pair with sharp, small blades and curved tips for better control and safety. These are particularly useful for maintaining shape between waxing or threading sessions. **Eyebrow razor offers** a quick and pain-free alternative to traditional plucking, particularly for shaping the edges of the brow or cleaning up peach fuzz around the area. However, they require a steady hand to avoid over-shaving.

Other useful tools include a **spoolie brush**, which is indispensable for combing and blending eyebrow hairs. A magnifying mirror ensures precision by offering a close-up view during the shaping process, and brow stencils can serve as a guide for those new to eyebrow shaping.

Selecting the Right Products: Powders, Pencils, Gels, and Pomades

While tools create the structure of your brows, the right products enhance their appearance. **Eyebrow powders** are ideal for filling sparse areas subtly, offering a soft, natural finish. These are best applied with an angled brush for precise application. On the other hand,

eyebrow pencils provide more control and definition. Opt for a pencil with a fine tip for mimicking individual hair strokes and a spoolie on the opposite end for blending.

Brow gels are perfect for taming unruly hairs and keeping them in place throughout the day. They come in clear formulas for a natural look or tinted options for added depth. **Eyebrow pomades** are highly pigmented and versatile, suitable for creating dramatic or bold eyebrow looks. These are particularly effective for individuals with sparse or uneven brows but require skill to avoid an overly drawn appearance.

When choosing products, it's important to consider your natural brow color, skin tone, and the desired intensity. Testing shades in natural light helps in achieving a seamless look. Investing in waterproof and long-lasting formulas ensures your eyebrows stay intact all day.

Hygiene and Maintenance of Tools

Proper hygiene and maintenance of your eyebrow tools are vital to prevent infections and ensure their longevity. Tweezers and scissors should be cleaned after every use with alcohol wipes to remove bacteria and residue. This step minimizes the risk of irritation or breakouts in the sensitive eyebrow area. For more thorough cleaning, soak tools in rubbing alcohol for a few minutes, then rinse and dry completely before storing them.

Eyebrow razors require extra care due to their direct contact with skin. Replace blades regularly to maintain sharpness and avoid using a dull blade, which can cause cuts or irritation. After use, rinse the razor under hot water to remove debris and pat it dry with a clean towel.

Spoolie brushes, angled brushes, and other applicators should be washed weekly using a gentle soap or brush cleaner. Regular cleaning removes product buildup and ensures smooth application. Store tools in a clean, dry environment, preferably in a dedicated case or pouch to protect them from dust and damage.

In addition to tool care, maintain hygiene during the grooming process by washing your hands thoroughly and disinfecting the brow area. This reduces the risk of transferring bacteria to the skin, helping to maintain healthy and well-groomed brows.

CHAPTER 3

PREPARING FOR EYEBROW SHAPING

Assessing Your Natural Brow Shape

Understanding your natural brow shape is the first and most crucial step in achieving perfectly shaped eyebrows. Your natural brow shape is determined by the natural arch, thickness, and direction of hair growth. To assess it accurately, start by observing your face in a well-lit mirror. Look for the high point of your arch, the beginning (closest to the nose), and the tail end of your brow. A simple way to determine proportions is by using the "golden ratio" method. Hold a straight object vertically against your nose to identify where your brow should begin, then angle it to pass through your iris to locate the arch, and finally angle it towards the outer corner of your eye to find the tail.

Pay attention to the symmetry of your brows, but keep in mind that eyebrows are sisters, not twins—they don't need to be identical but should appear balanced. Identify areas with sparse hair or overgrowth to guide your shaping process. Note the thickness of your brows as well; thicker brows are versatile and can be shaped easily, while thinner brows may require a lighter touch to avoid removing too much hair.

Skin Preparation: Cleansing and Softening Techniques

Proper skin preparation ensures a smoother and safer eyebrow-shaping experience while minimizing irritation and redness. Begin by cleansing the skin around your brows to remove makeup, oils, and dirt. Use a gentle facial cleanser or micellar water to avoid leaving any residue. This step helps prevent clogged pores and reduces the risk of infections.

After cleansing, soften the skin to make hair removal less painful. Soak a clean washcloth in warm water and apply it to your brows for 2-3 minutes. This process opens the pores, making the hair easier to remove. If you're using a threading or waxing method, consider applying a pre-wax or pre-threading gel, which can further soften the skin and create a barrier to protect it from irritation. For tweezing, you can gently exfoliate the area beforehand to remove dead skin cells and loosen ingrown hairs.

Tips for Minimizing Pain During Shaping

Pain is a common concern during eyebrow shaping, but several strategies can make the process more comfortable. If tweezing is your chosen method, ensure you use a high-quality pair of tweezers with a slanted tip for precision and reduced discomfort. Always pull the skin taut with one hand while tweezing with the other, as this minimizes tugging and reduces pain.

For waxing, test the wax temperature on your wrist to prevent burns and apply wax strips in the direction of hair growth. Pull the strip off quickly and close to the skin to minimize pain. Threading can be less painful when done on clean, dry skin; avoid applying any lotions beforehand, as this can cause slipping and irritation.

If you have a low pain threshold, consider using numbing creams designed for sensitive skin. Apply the cream about 20 minutes before shaping to allow it to take effect. Ice can also help; simply hold an ice cube wrapped in a cloth against your brows before and after shaping to reduce pain and inflammation. Finally, avoid shaping during your menstrual cycle, as pain sensitivity tends to be heightened during this time.

CHAPTER 4

EYEBROW SHAPING TECHNIQUES

Tweezing: Step-by-Step Guide for Precision Shaping

Tweezing is one of the most precise techniques for eyebrow shaping, allowing you to remove individual hairs for a polished look. Start by selecting a high-quality tweezer with a slanted or pointed tip for optimal grip. Begin by washing your face with warm water or placing a warm compress over your brows to open the pores and soften hair follicles, reducing discomfort.

Using a spoolie brush, comb your brows upward to see their natural shape and identify stray hairs. Work in good lighting and, if possible, use a magnifying mirror for precision. Hold your skin taut with one hand and pluck hairs in the direction of growth to prevent breakage and irritation. Begin tweezing from the bottom of the brow, working from the inner corner toward the arch and outward to the tail. Avoid over-plucking, focusing only on stray hairs outside your desired shape. Take regular breaks to assess symmetry and prevent over-shaping.

To finish, apply a soothing gel or aloe vera to calm the skin and reduce redness. With consistent practice, tweezing becomes an easy and effective way to maintain beautifully shaped brows.

Trimming: Maintaining Length and Tidiness

Trimming is essential for maintaining a polished appearance and controlling the length of eyebrow hairs. Start by gathering your tools: a spoolie brush and small, sharp scissors designed specifically for eyebrow trimming. Begin by brushing your brow hairs upward with the spoolie. This allows you to see which hairs extend beyond the natural brow shape.

Using your scissors, carefully trim the excess length of hairs that stick out, ensuring you cut one small section at a time. Avoid cutting too much at once, as overly short hairs can create unevenness. For best results, follow the natural curve of your brow while trimming. Afterward, brush the hairs downward and repeat the process for the lower brow line.

Trimming should be performed sparingly—every few weeks or when brows appear unruly. This technique is a quick way to enhance tidiness without altering the overall shape of your eyebrows.

Shaving: When and How to Use Brow Razors

Shaving with brow razors is a quick and painless method to remove fine hairs and clean up the brow area. It is best suited for people who want to maintain brow shape without removing significant amounts of hair. Before you begin, cleanse your skin and apply a thin layer of facial oil or shaving gel to reduce friction and prevent irritation.

Hold the brow razor at a 45-degree angle and gently glide it over the area you want to clean up. Avoid pressing too hard, as this can lead to nicks or cuts. Focus on removing stray hairs around the perimeter of your brows, especially on the upper brow bone and between the brows. Avoid shaping the brow's inner structure with a razor, as this can lead to unevenness.

After shaving, rinse your skin with cool water and apply a calming moisturizer. Remember that shaving does not provide as long-lasting results as tweezing or waxing, so it may need to be repeated more frequently.

Mapping Your Brows: Finding the Perfect Start, Arch, and End

Mapping your brows is a crucial step to achieving a well-balanced and flattering eyebrow shape. The process involves identifying three key points: the start of your brow, the arch, and the tail. Begin by holding a straight tool, such as a pencil or makeup brush, vertically against the side of your nose. The point where the tool intersects your brow marks the ideal starting point. This alignment helps create symmetry and opens up your eyes.

To find the arch, angle the tool from the side of your nose through the center of your iris. The spot where the tool meets your brow is where the highest point of your arch should be. This point adds definition and lifts your overall facial appearance. Finally, locate the tail by angling the tool from the side of your nose to the outer corner of your eye. The brow tail should end where the tool intersects your brow.

Once you've mapped these points, use an eyebrow pencil or powder to outline the ideal shape. This guide will make it easier to tweeze, trim, or shape your brows with precision. Mapping is particularly helpful for beginners and ensures that your brows complement your face shape.

CHAPTER 5

WAXING AND THREADING BASICS

Overview of Waxing: Tools, Techniques, and Precautions

Waxing is a popular hair removal method that provides a smooth and long-lasting finish. It works by removing hair from the root, which delays regrowth compared to shaving. For DIY eyebrow shaping, waxing can be an efficient way to clean up stray hairs and define the brow shape.

Tools Required: Basic tools for waxing include a high-quality eyebrow waxing kit, which typically contains soft or hard wax, applicator sticks, and muslin strips (for soft wax). A brow brush, tweezers for touch-ups, and a small pair of scissors can also come in handy. It's crucial to invest in products designed for sensitive facial skin to avoid irritation.

Techniques: Start by warming the wax according to the instructions provided in your kit. Clean the brow area to remove oil and makeup, then brush the brows into place. Apply the wax in the direction of hair growth using a small applicator stick. Place the strip over the wax (if using soft wax), press it down firmly, and then quickly pull it off in the opposite direction of hair growth. Hard wax doesn't require strips and should be peeled off after it hardens. Always wax in small sections to maintain precision.

Precautions: Be cautious not to over-apply wax or remove too much hair. Test the wax temperature on the back of your hand to avoid burns. If you're new to waxing, outline the desired brow shape with a white pencil to guide your application. Avoid waxing over cuts, pimples, or irritated skin. Patch testing the wax on a small area of skin is recommended for allergy prevention.

Threading: Mastering the Art for Clean Lines

Threading is a precise and natural method of hair removal that has been practiced for centuries. It involves using a cotton or polyester thread to pluck hairs in a clean, sharp line, making it ideal for eyebrow shaping.

Getting Started: All you need for threading is a strong piece of thread, a mirror, and steady hands. Trim the thread to about 12–18 inches, then tie it into a loop. Hold the loop taut and twist it several times to create a central knot. This twisted section is what traps and pulls the hair out.

Technique: Sit in front of a well-lit mirror and hold one end of the thread loop in each hand, creating a triangle shape. Place the twisted section against the brow area where you want to remove hair. Open and close the loop with your fingers to move the twists back and forth, catching hairs and pulling them out from the root. Work in small sections for control and precision.

Advantages of Threading: Threading allows for incredibly clean lines, making it perfect for shaping arches. It doesn't involve heat or chemicals, making it a good option for sensitive skin. While threading may require some practice, it is cost-effective and offers professional results.

Safety and Aftercare for Waxing and Threading

Proper safety measures and aftercare are essential to prevent irritation, ingrown hairs, and infections after waxing or threading.

Before the Procedure: Ensure your tools are clean and sanitized. For waxing, exfoliate the brow area a day before to remove dead skin cells, which helps the wax adhere better. Avoid applying heavy creams or oils on the day of the procedure, as they can interfere with hair removal.

Immediate Aftercare: After waxing, apply a soothing gel or lotion containing aloe vera or witch hazel to calm the skin. Avoid touching the brow area with unwashed hands, as this can introduce bacteria to freshly opened pores. For threading, gently cleanse the area with a mild toner or antiseptic to reduce the risk of irritation.

Long-term Care: Avoid direct sun exposure, hot showers, and saunas for at least 24 hours after waxing or threading to prevent inflammation. Refrain from using exfoliating products or makeup on the brows for a day or two. To prevent ingrown hairs, exfoliate the area gently a few days after the procedure.

Signs of Complications: Watch for redness, swelling, or bumps lasting more than a day, as these could indicate an allergic reaction or infection. If symptoms persist, consult a dermatologist.

By following these tips and maintaining a consistent routine, you can ensure your brows remain well-groomed and your skin stays healthy.

CHAPTER 6

FILLING AND ENHANCING EYEBROWS

Techniques for Natural-Looking Fills

Achieving natural-looking filled eyebrows involves mastering techniques that mimic the appearance of real hair. Start by selecting a fine-tipped brow pencil or a brow pen designed for precision. Use light, hair-like strokes to fill in sparse areas, ensuring the lines follow the natural growth direction of your eyebrow hairs. Avoid harsh, heavy lines, as they can make the brows look unnatural and drawn on. Instead, aim for a soft gradient effect by concentrating more pigment on the sparse areas and blending outward for a seamless finish.

Another effective technique is the use of a brow pomade with an angled brush. Dip the brush lightly into the product, tapping off any excess, and outline the shape of your brows before filling in. This method allows for better control and a more defined shape while still looking natural. For added realism, consider combining two shades—one lighter for the front of the brows and a slightly darker one for the tails. This creates dimension and enhances the overall natural appearance of your brows.

Choosing the Right Color and Formula for Your Brows

The key to perfectly filled brows lies in selecting the right color and formula. Start by identifying your brow's undertone—cool, warm, or neutral—and choose a shade that complements your natural hair color. For a natural look, opt for a brow product that is one to two shades lighter than your hair color if you are dark-haired, and one to two shades darker if you are light-haired. Avoid overly dark or ashy shades, as they can appear harsh or unnatural.

Formulas play a critical role in the outcome. Brow pencils are versatile and ideal for precise filling and shaping. Brow powders offer a softer, more diffused look, making them suitable for those who prefer subtle enhancement. Pomades provide a bolder, defined appearance and are best for those with sparse or uneven brows. Gels, especially tinted ones, are perfect for setting the brows in place while adding a hint of color and volume. Testing different formulas and shades is essential to find the one that works best for your unique brows.

Enhancing Volume and Texture with Brow Gels and Powders

Brow gels and powders are excellent tools for adding volume and texture to your eyebrows. Start by brushing your brows upward with a spoolie to reveal their natural shape and identify sparse areas. Use a tinted brow gel to add color and volume, brushing in short, upward strokes. This technique not only enhances the brow's fullness but also sets the hair in place for a polished look. Fiber-infused gels are particularly effective for creating a thickened appearance, as they adhere to the hairs and add a natural, feathery texture.

For a soft, textured look, brow powders can be applied using a small, angled brush. Dab the brush into the powder, tap off the excess, and gently sweep it over the brows, focusing on areas that need filling. Powders blend effortlessly and are ideal for creating a soft gradient effect, especially when combined with brow gels. To finish, use a clear brow gel to lock everything in place and add a subtle sheen, giving your brows a well-groomed, voluminous appearance.

CHAPTER 7

MAINTAINING YOUR EYEBROWS

Daily Care Routines for Healthy Brows

Healthy eyebrows require consistent care to stay well-groomed and lush. Incorporating a simple yet effective daily routine can make a significant difference. Start by cleansing your brows gently during your skincare routine. Use a mild, sulfate-free cleanser to remove dirt, oil, and makeup residue. Clean brows promote hair growth and prevent clogged hair follicles that can lead to thinning. Pat them dry with a soft towel to avoid tugging on the delicate skin around your brows.

Moisturizing your brows is equally important. Apply a lightweight, non-comedogenic moisturizer or a brow serum infused with nourishing ingredients such as biotin, peptides, or castor oil. These not only hydrate the brow area but also stimulate hair growth. Brushing your brows daily with a spoolie brush helps distribute natural oils evenly while keeping the hairs neat and tangle-free.

For added protection, apply sunscreen over your brows to shield them from UV damage, which can weaken brow hairs. If you use makeup, choose products specifically designed for brows, such as brow pencils or gels, as they are gentler and less likely to irritate. Lastly, avoid touching your brows throughout the day to prevent transferring dirt and bacteria that could lead to breakouts or infections.

Tips for Preventing Over-Plucking

Over-plucking is a common mistake that can lead to sparse and uneven brows. To avoid this, always start by identifying your brow's natural shape. Use a brow mapping technique by aligning a pencil vertically along the side of your nose to find where your brow should begin, and then angle it toward the outer corner of your eye to find the tail. Mark these points lightly with a brow pencil for guidance before plucking.

Invest in a quality pair of tweezers with a slanted tip for precise removal. Never use magnifying mirrors as they can cause you to over-focus on small areas and pluck excessively. Instead, use a standard mirror in good lighting to maintain perspective.

Adopt the "less is more" approach by plucking only stray hairs outside your natural brow line. It's best to tweeze after a shower when your pores are open, making hair removal easier and less painful. Additionally, take breaks while shaping your brows to assess symmetry and avoid impulsive over-plucking. Remember, regular grooming every few weeks is better than attempting to perfect your brows daily.

Managing Unruly or Sparse Areas

Unruly or sparse brows require special attention to achieve a polished look. For unruly brows, start by trimming long or stray hairs. Use small, sharp scissors and a spoolie to comb the hairs upward, snipping only the tips to avoid over-cutting. Set unruly hairs in place using a clear or tinted brow gel, brushing in the direction of hair growth.

Sparse areas can be filled using makeup products like brow pencils, powders, or pomades. Choose a shade that closely matches your natural brow color for a seamless finish. Use light, feathery strokes to mimic natural hair, concentrating on areas with the most gaps. A brow stencil can also help achieve consistent results.

For a more long-term solution, consider using brow growth serums with proven ingredients like peptides, keratin, or panthenol to stimulate growth in sparse areas. Alternatively, natural remedies like applying castor oil or aloe vera can be beneficial over time.

If you struggle with brow asymmetry or significant sparsity, professional treatments like microblading or brow lamination can help achieve a fuller and more uniform appearance. Regular maintenance and patience are key to managing unruly or sparse brows effectively.

CHAPTER 8

CORRECTING COMMON EYEBROW ISSUES

Dealing with Uneven Eyebrows

Uneven eyebrows are one of the most common beauty concerns and can result from natural asymmetry, over-plucking, or improper shaping techniques. The first step in correcting uneven eyebrows is assessing the natural shape and structure of your brows. Stand in front of a mirror with good lighting and examine both brows closely. Use a brow pencil or ruler to measure the alignment of the start, arch, and tail of each brow. The inner corners of the brows should align with the bridge of the nose, and the arch should peak just above the outer edge of the iris.

To even out the brows, start by filling in the sparser or lower brow using a brow pencil, pomade, or powder that matches your natural hair color. Use light, feathery strokes to mimic the appearance of hair and create a balanced look. For the higher or thicker brow, avoid over-filling and focus on subtly matching its fullness and shape to the other. If necessary, trim or pluck stray hairs beneath the fuller brow to make it match the other. Always use small, measured adjustments to avoid over-compensating.

If symmetry is challenging to achieve, consider using stencils or a brow mapping technique. This involves marking key points on your face to guide shaping and filling. For those new to DIY brow shaping, consulting a professional once for guidance can help establish a symmetrical baseline you can maintain at home.

Fixing Over-Plucked or Thinning Brows

Over-plucked or thinning brows can drastically change the appearance of your face, but with patience and the right techniques, they can be restored. First, avoid plucking or waxing entirely for a few weeks to allow natural regrowth. During this time, nourish your brow area with products containing castor oil, vitamin E, or peptides, which can stimulate hair growth and strengthen existing strands.

In the meantime, fill in sparse areas using a brow pencil or powder. Choose a shade that closely matches your natural brow color and use short, upward strokes to mimic natural hair growth. Avoid creating harsh lines, as a softer look appears more natural.

If regrowth is slow or patchy, consider applying a brow serum designed to promote growth. These products are often enriched with keratin or biotin, which can help enhance the thickness and density of your brows over time. If you're struggling with shaping during regrowth, let your brows grow fully before consulting a professional for reshaping.

Solutions for Patchy or Bald Spots

Patchy or bald spots in eyebrows can result from genetics, over-plucking, or conditions like alopecia. Addressing these issues starts with identifying the cause. If the issue is medical, consulting a dermatologist may be necessary to treat underlying conditions.

For cosmetic solutions, brow makeup is a reliable and immediate fix. A waterproof brow pencil or powder works well to fill in gaps. Use small, light strokes to mimic hair growth, paying extra attention to blending for a seamless look. Brow gels with fibers can add volume and give the illusion of fuller brows in sparse areas.

Consider microblading or brow tattooing for a long-term solution. These semi-permanent cosmetic procedures involve depositing pigment under the skin to simulate the appearance of natural hair. While these treatments can be costly, they provide a low-maintenance solution for addressing severe gaps or bald spots.

Natural remedies, such as massaging the brow area with castor oil or aloe vera gel, can promote blood circulation and stimulate regrowth. Additionally, incorporating a diet rich in biotin, omega-3 fatty acids, and vitamin E can support hair health. Patience and consistency are key, as hair regrowth takes time and care.

CHAPTER 9

EYEBROW TRENDS AND STYLES

Exploring Popular Eyebrow Shapes Through the Years

Eyebrow trends have evolved significantly over the decades, reflecting societal changes and beauty ideals. In the 1920s, thin, dramatically arched brows dominated the scene, influenced by silent film stars who favored a pencil-thin look to convey emotion. This trend carried into the 1930s but with a softer, more rounded arch. The 1940s introduced a slightly thicker and more natural style, as women opted for groomed brows with a defined arch to frame their faces.

The 1950s marked the era of the bold brow, with icons like Audrey Hepburn and Elizabeth Taylor setting the standard. Women embraced fuller, darker brows, often accentuated with makeup to achieve a polished look. By the 1960s, the pendulum swung back toward thinner brows, but this time paired with a high, defined arch to complement the modern fashion era. The 1970s brought a natural aesthetic, with minimal grooming reflecting the bohemian spirit of the decade.

The 1990s and early 2000s revived the pencil-thin brow, often heavily plucked or waxed into sharp arches. However, this trend was later criticized for its damaging effects, leading to the resurgence of fuller, more natural brows in the 2010s, spearheaded by celebrities like Cara Delevingne. Today, eyebrow styles are as diverse as ever, ranging from fluffy, laminated brows to sleek, microbladed perfection, allowing individuals to express their unique style.

Adapting Trends to Suit Your Face Shape

While trends offer inspiration, tailoring eyebrow styles to your unique face shape ensures the most flattering look. For round faces, a high, well-defined arch can add length and dimension, balancing the soft features. Square faces benefit from gently curved brows that soften the angular jawline, while heart-shaped faces look best with slightly rounded brows to complement their tapered chin.

Oval faces are versatile and can pull off a variety of eyebrow styles, but a soft arch that follows the natural brow line is universally flattering. For long faces, flat, straight brows help create the illusion of width, balancing facial proportions. Diamond-shaped faces should consider softer, rounded brows to reduce the prominence of angular features.

When adapting trends, it's essential to consider eyebrow thickness, length, and placement relative to your eyes and nose. Consulting a professional or using a stencil can help achieve symmetry and alignment. By customizing trendy styles to your face shape, you enhance your natural beauty while staying current.

Natural vs. Bold Looks: Finding Your Style

Choosing between natural and bold eyebrow styles depends on your personality, lifestyle, and beauty preferences. Natural brows emphasize simplicity and ease, celebrating minimal grooming and the unique growth pattern of your brows. This style often involves subtle shaping, light trimming, and minimal use of makeup, allowing your face to appear fresh and youthful.

In contrast, bold brows command attention and often involve the use of products like pomades, powders, or pencils to enhance fullness and definition. This style suits individuals who enjoy experimenting with dramatic makeup looks or want their brows to be a focal point. Bold brows can range from structured and sharp to fluffy and feathery, offering versatility.

To find your style, consider the occasions you're preparing for and the time you can dedicate to maintenance. A natural look is perfect for everyday wear and those seeking a low-maintenance routine, while bold brows work well for events, photoshoots, or individuals with a flair for dramatic aesthetics. Experimenting with different shapes, shades, and techniques will help you discover the perfect balance between natural elegance and bold beauty.

CHAPTER 10

LONG-TERM BROW CARE AND GROWTH

Setting Realistic Expectations for Hair Growth and Health

When embarking on a DIY eyebrow shaping and maintenance routine, it is essential to set realistic expectations for the growth and overall health of your eyebrow hairs. Unlike scalp hair, which typically grows at a consistent rate, eyebrow hairs grow at a slower pace and can be more prone to thinning due to various factors such as age, genetics, and hormonal changes. On average, eyebrow hair grows at a rate of about 0.16 mm per day, which means it can take weeks or even months to see noticeable growth if you're trying to restore over-plucked or sparse eyebrows.

It's also important to remember that eyebrow hair growth is cyclical, with each hair going through a shedding phase. Even if you diligently follow a hair growth regimen, it's natural for some hairs to fall out as part of this cycle. Therefore, patience is critical in the process. Setting achievable goals based on your current brow condition will help you avoid frustration. For instance, if your goal is to regrow fuller brows, expect the process to take several months, depending on the individual's hair growth cycle. Moreover, it is essential to consider that not all eyebrow hairs may grow back the same way. Factors such as the texture and color of the new growth may differ from the existing hairs, leading to an uneven appearance, which can be corrected over time with proper shaping.

Additionally, maintaining healthy brows isn't solely about growing them; it's about ensuring they remain strong and vibrant. Just as with scalp hair, the health of your eyebrows is influenced by your diet, skincare routine, and how well you protect them from damage. Using too many harsh products or over-tweezing can slow down hair regeneration and affect the health of existing brow hairs. Understanding these factors and adjusting your expectations to the natural rhythm of hair growth can ensure a more positive and manageable brow care journey.

Combining Natural Remedies with Healthy Lifestyle Practices

One of the best ways to enhance eyebrow growth and maintain their health is to incorporate natural remedies alongside healthy lifestyle practices. While there's no magical solution for instantly thickening your brows, using natural oils and serums can help nourish the follicles, stimulate growth, and prevent damage. Castor oil, for example, is widely known for its high content of ricinoleic acid, which promotes hair growth. Applying a small amount of castor oil to your brows every night with a clean spoolie brush can keep the hairs moisturized, thereby reducing breakage and encouraging thicker, healthier growth.

Along with natural remedies, incorporating healthy lifestyle habits is essential for long-term brow health. A balanced diet rich in vitamins and minerals plays a vital role in the growth and overall strength of your hair. Nutrients such as vitamin E, biotin, omega-3 fatty acids, and zinc are essential for promoting healthy hair follicles. Foods such as nuts, leafy greens, eggs, and fish are great additions to your diet to boost eyebrow health. Additionally, staying hydrated is crucial, as dehydration can lead to brittle and weak hair. Drinking enough water helps to keep your skin and hair hydrated, promoting optimal growth conditions for your eyebrows.

Sleep also plays a critical role in the regeneration of hair cells, so ensure that you are getting 7-8 hours of sleep per night to support overall hair health. Minimizing stress is equally important, as high levels of stress can contribute to hair loss, including thinning eyebrows. Engaging in activities such as yoga, meditation, or simply taking time to relax can reduce stress and prevent eyebrow thinning caused by tension or anxiety. By combining natural remedies with healthy lifestyle practices, you are creating an environment conducive to healthy and sustained eyebrow growth.

Holistic Habits for Healthy, Lustrous Hair

Maintaining long-term eyebrow health requires more than just external treatments; holistic habits should become a core part of your routine to promote luster and strength in your eyebrows. Taking a comprehensive approach means focusing on both external care and internal well-being. Start by practicing gentle eyebrow care to avoid unnecessary damage. Avoid over-plucking, threading, or waxing, as these methods can weaken the hair follicles over time, hindering growth. Instead, opt for trimming and tweezing with caution, ensuring that you only remove stray hairs to maintain the natural shape of your brows.

In addition to careful grooming, consider massaging your brows to stimulate blood flow to the hair follicles. Gently massaging your eyebrows using oils like olive oil or jojoba oil helps to nourish and invigorate the area, promoting faster growth. A small amount of pressure applied during the massage can also activate the sebaceous glands, producing natural oils that help protect your brow hair and skin from dryness.

Furthermore, it's important to manage the external factors that can impact eyebrow health, such as excessive exposure to sun or harsh weather conditions. UV rays and environmental pollutants can cause hair damage, so be sure to protect your brows by wearing hats or using products with SPF. The skin around your eyebrows can also benefit from moisturizing, which helps maintain skin elasticity and prevents dry, flaky patches that may inhibit healthy hair growth.

Lastly, incorporate stress management into your daily life. High levels of stress can contribute to a variety of hair problems, including thinning eyebrows. Engaging in activities that promote relaxation, such as exercise, mindfulness, and deep breathing, can help reduce cortisol levels and support healthy hair growth. By embracing these holistic habits, you will create a sustainable routine that promotes not only the health of your eyebrows but also your overall well-being.

Troubleshooting and Adjusting Your Routine Over Time

As you progress in your DIY eyebrow shaping and maintenance journey, it's essential to stay flexible and adjust your routine based on the results you observe. Not all brow growth methods will work the same way for everyone, and the effectiveness of your approach may change over time. Therefore, troubleshooting and making adjustments to your routine can ensure you are continuously working toward achieving the best possible results.

If you're not seeing the desired results, first assess whether your expectations were realistic from the start. Are you expecting a fuller look too quickly, or have you allowed sufficient time for the natural growth cycle to take its course? If you've been following a specific routine for several weeks without noticeable improvement, it may be worth experimenting with other natural remedies, such as switching oils or incorporating different vitamins and supplements into your diet. For example, if castor oil is not working for you, try using rosemary or coconut oil, both of which are known for their hair-stimulating properties.

On the other hand, if your brows appear too sparse after attempting regrowth, it might indicate that your tweezing or grooming habits were too aggressive in the past. In such cases, it's important to give your brows a break, stop plucking or waxing for a few weeks, and allow them time to recover. It may also be helpful to map out your brow shape using eyebrow pencils or stencils to guide your grooming process, ensuring that you're not overdoing it or removing more hair than necessary.

Adjusting your lifestyle habits can also play a role in troubleshooting. If you've been following a healthy diet but are still experiencing sparse or thinning brows, consider revisiting your food choices and supplements. Sometimes, it may take more time to see changes in hair growth, and in some cases, you may need to increase your intake of certain vitamins or minerals. Additionally, monitor the impact of stress and other environmental factors on your hair growth, and adjust your habits accordingly.

In conclusion, adjusting your routine over time allows you to fine-tune your approach to eyebrow care. By staying patient, being open to change, and troubleshooting when necessary, you can continue to improve your results and achieve healthier, fuller brows.

www.ingramcontent.com/pod-product-compliance
Lightning Source LLC
Chambersburg PA
CBHW061307250726
48653CB00002B/817